IT'S ONLY A HEADACHE

The Cluster Headache Handbook

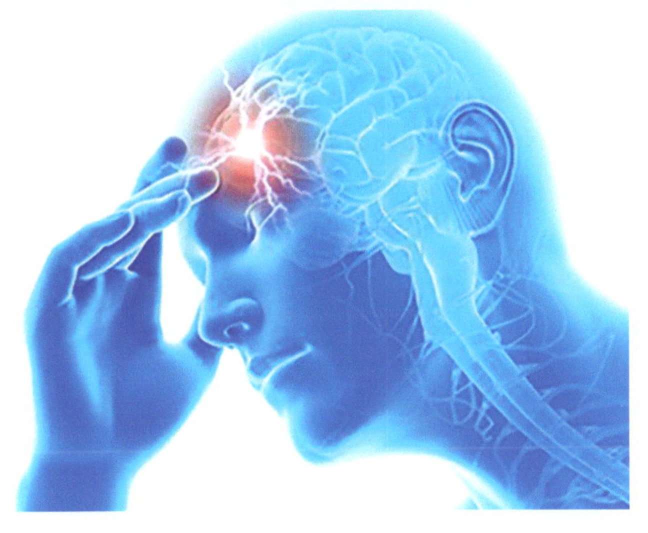

Jack Boyd

This book is dedicated to each and every cluster headache sufferer who has ever lived.

Table of Contents

Introduction

At the time of this writing, I am 74 years old, 5'10" tall, 175 lbs. and in excellent health. I have never had a heart attack or a stroke, have never had cancer and am not on any medications. **I have also had cluster headaches since the age of 21**. I come to this project very reluctantly for many of the same reasons I did not like to speak about my clusters during these 53 years. Who could possibly understand? As I have often said, if I didn't have this bizarre condition called cluster headaches, I wouldn't believe they existed. But exist they do.

For those looking for some magic bullet, as in drink lots of water or find Jesus and your clusters will go away this will not be the right book for you. In fact, this handbook won't be much of a handbook at all. I will offer sober truths and humbly share my experiences, for cluster headaches are indeed humbling. There will be no breast beating as in how I beat clusters and you can do it too. My experience as someone with 50 plus years of episodic cluster headaches is informative only in that my experience is not revelatory but rather typical.

And perhaps most importantly, be skeptical of anything I write. I am neither a doctor nor a scientist and whatever you do, get professional guidance from a doctor, preferably a neurologist. I will refrain from suggesting medications or treatments but rather offer what the research and data provide and what has worked for me. And if I speculate about anything I will be sure to state that. I will also refrain from writing about chronic cluster headaches, a subset of clusters that thankfully I have no experience with. I will attempt to compile the best information available about clusters in a simple, readable, handy format.

I can't **help** but write this book and I know you will forgive me for doing so.

The Diagnosis

It is not a bad idea to explain how cluster headaches are diagnosed before we go any further. They **cannot** be diagnosed through a blood test or a test of any other bodily fluids. An MRI or an x-ray is of no value. There simply is no reliable physical examination that can be definitive. So, what does that leave? A careful description of symptoms presented to a health care professional (preferably a neurologist) with an intimate and extensive understanding of cluster headaches.

So, what exactly are those symptoms? Well thankfully they are very discreet and unmistakable and are as follows:

- **Excruciating pain centered behind one eye**

- **A red droopy eye lid**

- **A stuffed nose**

- **Lacrimation (tearing)**

- **Pain that lasts for an hour or two, vanishes and then returns hours or days later.**

- **Restlessness***

***Restlessness may be a distinguishing characteristic for clusters. Unlike other vascular or neuro-vascular headaches, such as migraine, one cannot just sleep it off. And most importantly do not self-diagnose or self-medicate. Go to a specialist if you suspect you have clusters.**

Cluster Headache Facts

Incidence - .1 % (1 out of 1,000) of the population

Men are 2.5 times to 3 times more likely to have clusters

88 percent of those diagnosed with clusters smoke cigarettes

14 to 39 times more likely to have clusters if they have a 1st-degree relative who also had cluster headaches

Chronic cluster headaches are defined as one year or more without remission

Higher incidence is also reported in patients with a history of head trauma

[1]

---

[1] https://www.ncbi.nlm.nih.gov/books/NBK544241/

My Life With Clusters

(Anecdotal evidence is not without value)

It was 1971 and this 21-year-old was awakened from sleep on his mother's living room pull-out couch early in the morning with an excruciating headache the likes of which I had never experienced before. Centered behind my right eye, it was accompanied by tearing, a stuffy nose and a red droopy lid. It lasted about an hour or two. I thought that I had gotten my head stuck in the frame overnight and this might be a reason for the headache. After the headache returned on the next day and the day after that and the day after that, I thought it wise to go to the doctor. His diagnosis was a sinus infection, and he prescribed an anti-biotic (the mother of all overly prescribed medications) and a pain reliever, the name of which I do not recall. He asked me very few questions and as I recall there was no bacterial swab. Needless to say, these medications had no effect.

The prevalence of cluster headaches is approximately 1 in 1,000[2] and the ratio of men to women is 2.5 to 1. This initial doctor's visit was with a general practitioner who may have never had a cluster headache patient in his life, and I am more than willing to concede that I may have done a poor job in describing my symptoms. I accepted his sinus infection diagnosis and employed all the stoicism I could muster to get through this sinus infection. My first cycle with clusters lasted about 4 or 5 weeks and went away as suddenly as it appeared. So, the next several

---

[2] Epub 2008 Apr 16.

The incidence and prevalence of cluster headache: a meta-analysis of population-based studies

M Fischera 1, M Marziniak, I Gralow, S Evers

years were my bogus sinus infection period, a period where I coped by knowing each bout of sinus infection (clusters) would end in due time. I can still cringe, however, all these years later when I recall friends rolling their eyes when I said I couldn't play touch football that day because I had a sinus infection. And then about six years later the most remarkable thing happened. It was one of those defining events that seem to become even more important in retrospect. I was thumbing through a magazine when I saw a health column, and something caught my eye. That something was a description of cluster headaches that matched exactly what I had. **This thing had a name!! Excruciating pain always behind one eye, tearing stuffed nose, red droopy eye lid, bouts of one or two hours that came in episodes of 4 to 5 weeks.** I must admit that I was a little disappointed in the name then and I remain disappointed in the name now. One might think that a condition widely considered to be one of the most painful known to man would have a more compelling name. But more about branding later when we address the history of clusters.

Naturally, as you might imagine, I got my hands on anything I could find regarding the literature on cluster headaches. My interest centered on two things – would I outgrow them and are they associated with any other maladies? This news was both good and bad. The bad news was that although it was likely I would eventually outgrow them, they would probably last the better part of my lifetime. And as far as comorbidities were concerned, or to put it another way, were my clusters damaging me, the news was good. Despite some initial literature that implied that sufferers had disproportionate rates of heart disease, clusters are actually benign.[3] It seems that some of the initial

---

[3] J Headache Pain. 2017; 18(1): 76.

Published online 2017 Jul 24. doi: 10.1186/s10194-017-0785-3 The comorbidity burden of patients with cluster headache: a population-based study

studies did not control for rates of smoking and drinking. Cluster sufferers tend to smoke and drink heavily. When that behavior is controlled for, cluster sufferers have normal rates of heart disease. The initial news about heart disease led me to step up an already healthy lifestyle. Part of my approach to this condition was to get in the best shape I could to do battle with this monster.

The literature on treatment was more problematic. The literature clearly stated that pharmaceutical treatments included medicine with very strong and potentially damaging side effects. Studies also stated that cluster headaches do not in any way lend themselves to biofeedback as a treatment regimen. So, this purist (fool) opted to continue coping sans medication.

As I got older, and my employment responsibilities became more demanding I started to look for treatment. My first foray into treatment was to get my hands on oxygen which can work as an abortive. Inhaling pure oxygen at a rate of at least seven liters per minute for fifteen minutes is highly effective at stopping a cluster headache in its tracks and it worked fairly well for me.[4] Treatment can be categorized as abortive or preventative. Waiting for an attack to inhale pure oxygen is not particularly practical and can upset those in your workplace. In one of those moments of pure serendipity I finally sought preventative treatment when my employer scheduled me to give a speech in front of five hundred poor souls in Phoenix Arizona in 1988 while I was in an episode of clusters. The thought of an attack

---

[4] Oxygen treatment for cluster headache attacks at different flow rates: a double-blind, randomized, crossover study
- Thijs H. T. Dirkx,
- Danielle Y. P. Haane &
- Peter J. Koehler

The Journal of Headache and Pain volume 19, Article number: 94 (2018)

in front of that many people made me apoplectic. **So, I finally went to a neurologist who told me he had a new treatment that was highly effective as a preventative and this drug was called Verapamil. And it worked! I have been using it ever since.** [5] Verapamil is a calcium channel blocker commonly used for hypertension. Most neurologists consider it the drug of choice for episodic cluster prevention. The dose needed to prevent clusters can be large and for those with heart issues it can be contraindicated. My experience was that it works very well and the only side effect I experienced was constipation. I only take Verapamil when a cycle starts and when the cycle ends I stop. My neurologist once suggested that I take verapamil all the time. I thought that was poor advice and I filed that suggestion in my "be your own advocate" folder. Of course, this was the same neurologist who said that all of his cluster headache patients looked the same. I was afraid to ask what he meant by that just in case I would be disappointed by the answer. There are other abortives besides oxygen and there are other preventives besides verapamil. Do not even consider taking these meds without your doctor's approval and monitoring.

One of the more remarkable aspects of my cluster career is how the time between episodes has steadily grown. An episode once a year became every two years, then three years to my current nine years and counting. I am indeed outgrowing them albeit very gradually.

---

[5] What is the evidence for verapamil for prevention of cluster headache? Source UKMi · Published 19 October 2020Topics: Neurological disorders · Verapamil

The Painful History

The earliest reference to cluster headaches in the medical literature occurred in 1641 and was provided by the Dutch physician Nicolas Tulp. Cluster headaches have gone through numerous name changes over the years and these names include: erythroprosopalgia of Bing, ciliary neuralgia, migrainous neuralgia, erythromelagia of the head, Horton's headache, histaminic cephalalgia, petrosal neuralgia, sphenopalatine neuralgia, Vidian neuralgia, Sluder's neuralgia, sphenopalatine neuralgia. and hemicrania angioparalyticia. The current name of cluster headaches was provided in 1952 by the American physician E. Charles Kunkle. If given my druthers I would change the name of clusters to any of the previous iterations which seem to offer the gravitas that these headaches warrant. My current favorite might be erythroprosopalgia of Bing. Of course, attempts at pronunciation might bring on a headache.

It is generally considered that the most famous person to suffer from cluster headaches (besides you and I) might be Frank Capra, the highly successful and beloved Director who gave us ***It's A Wonderful Life*** among other great movies. Frank Capra's description of a cluster headache:

"Suddenly a huge phantom bird sank three talons of its angry claws deeply into my head and face and tried to lift me. No warnings, no preliminary signs. Just wham! A massive, killing pain came over my right eye. I clutched my head, stumbled out to the broad lawns and over the hedges to the deserted tennis courts and then, there in the dark, I moaned, I panted. Ballooned my cheeks, blew out short bursts of air, licked my hot lips, wiped tears that poured out of my right eye, and clawed at my head trying to uproot the fiendish talons from their iron grip.

One racking hour later the talons let go. The paroxysm eased as suddenly as it had convulsed. Euphoria set in. It's gone! Whopping headache, but it's gone!..."

My description of the pain would not be nearly as dramatic. I describe the pain as intense, boring and unrelenting accompanied by feelings of dread and an intense restlessness. Restlessness is a defining component of clusters which helps to distinguish them from migraines. Sufferers pace, they keep moving and there is no way they can sleep it off.

How painful are clusters? After all, pain is the most subjective of feelings. It takes a stimulus and a reaction to that stimulus. The reaction includes one's general tolerance for pain and their immediate emotional state. Comparing pain between conditions and diseases is a fraughtful enterprise but I will try nonetheless. Any study that I have ever read ranks cluster headaches among the most painful conditions known to man,. Propriety compels me to include this recent study by U.S. News and World Report that ranks it **among** the most painful. [6] And I have no doubt that I could cite several studies that rank cluster headaches at number one.

---

[5] Ranking The Most Painful Medical Conditions

Find out which medical conditions are ranked as the most painful, according to experts. Learn how these conditions are treated and what you can do to manage your pain.

By Christine Comizio

April 13, 2023, at 4:38 p.m. **U.S. News and World Report**

Triggers and Treatment

Triggers are understandably one of the more controversial and problematic aspects of clustering. The reasons for this are many but certainly includes these two considerations:

1 – Cause and effect is difficult to determine under the best of circumstances and it requires controlled scientific study. Clusters are rare and there are few scientific studies to be found.

2 – Other headaches, migraines and tension to name just two, have well documented triggers so why not Clusters?

Let me introduce a little personal perspective on this matter. One of the reasons I have always been reluctant to talk about my clusters was the impetus for the most well-meaning around me (including my family) to offer trigger advice. I am sure if one had queried my family regarding Jackie (my family name) and his headaches they might have offered something like this – "he gets headaches because he holds in his emotions" – YIKES!! One lady I worked with said I got headaches because I slept too much – Another YIKES!! No worries if I wasn't a cluster sufferer I am sure I might offer similar psychobabble.

So, are there well documented and accepted triggers? Yes there are. Alcohol is generally considered to be the most common trigger. Drink alcohol during an episode and it is likely to bring on a bout. I am a total teetotaler now and have been for many years but in my early twenties I drank occasionally. If I drank any alcohol at all during a cycle it would bring on an immediate attack. Smoking is generally considered to be another trigger and cluster headache sufferers smoke at a higher rate than the general population. I don't smoke so I have no personal experience with this as a trigger. I will not speculate on any other triggers but will suggest that triggers are often misunderstood and overstated. I should also note that most of my cluster attacks begin while I am sleeping. I have had more than my share of attacks during the day but most have woken me from a deep sleep.

As stated earlier, treatments are either abortive or preventive. I have experience with only two – oxygen as an abortive and verapamil as a preventative. I have no experience with any other treatments and I will refrain offering any insights. These are the most commonly used treatments:

Abortives – please note that all drugs have side effects and this list is no exception. No one should take any drug without a prescription and full knowledge of the risks.

Oxygen	Breathing in pure oxygen
Triptans - Sumatriptan **(Imitrex)**	Injections or nose spray
Octreotide (Sandostatin)	Injection
Local anesthetics (Lidocaine)	Administered through nose
Dihydroergotamine	Administered through a vein

Preventatives – please note that all drugs have side effects and this list is no exception. No one should take any drug without a prescription and full knowledge of the risks.

Calcium channel blockers (Verapamil, Calan, Verelan)	Daily pills
Corticosteroids (prednisone)	Pills
Galcanezumab (Emgality)	Monthly injection
Lithium	Pills
Noninvasive vagus nerve stimulation (VNS).	Electrical stimulation to the vagus nerve through the skin
Nerve block	Injection of pain relieving medicine into the back of the head

Cluster headaches are not easily treatable and often call for powerful medication. Every drug listed here has side effects and no one should take any of these drugs without a physician's oversight and full knowledge of the side effects and risks.

The Physiology

It is probably no surprise to anyone with the least bit of familiarity with cluster headaches that the physiology related to clusters is both poorly understood and amazingly complex. And the best place to start is to understand the hypothalamus, that most basic and primitive part of our brain.

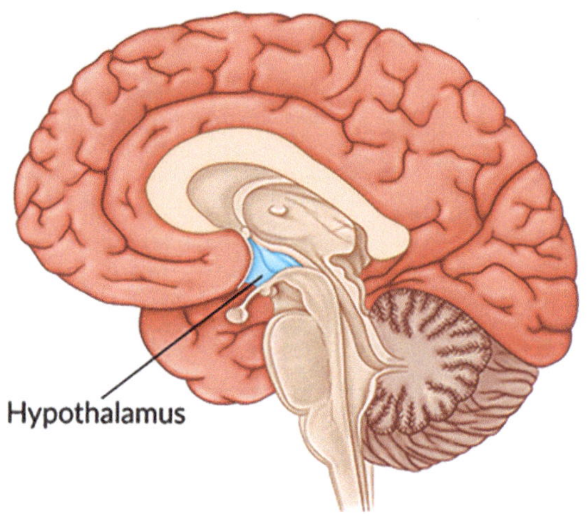

The hypothalamus is located deep inside our brains and controls our most basic bodily functions. It controls our autonomic nervous systems and manages our hormones. And it is strongly implicated as a root cause of clusters. Numerous studies have concluded that hypothalamus activity is abnormal during a cluster attack.[7] The hypothalamus regulates circadian rhythms and may be responsible for the seasonal aspect of clusters.

---

7 https://www.mountsinai.org/health-library/report/headaches-cluster

"Cluster headache is a **neurovascular** rather than a **vascular** headache, with vascular cerebral changes being driven by the effects of trigeminal-autonomic reflex activation."[8] I consider this to be the most salient description of the physiology of a cluster headache - **neurovascular** indeed. The principal nerve involved is the trigeminal nerve, the largest of the 12 cranial nerves in our brains.

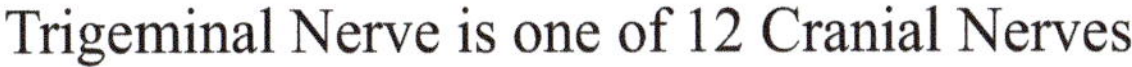

Trigeminal Nerve is one of 12 Cranial Nerves

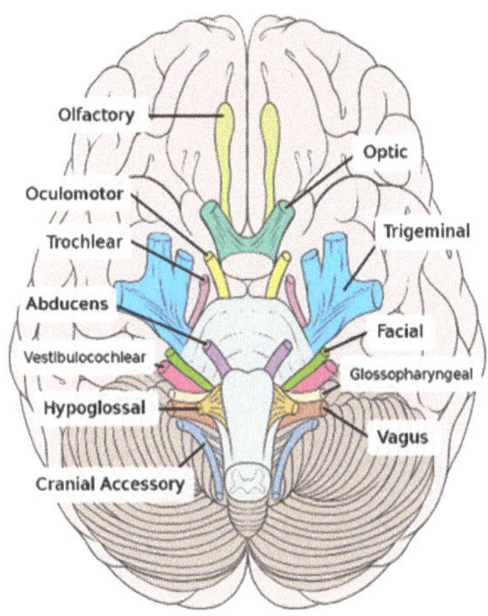

At the risk of oversimplification, a cluster attack involves inflammation of the trigeminal nerve which, in turn, stimulates the autonomic system causing cluster headache symptoms such as eye tearing and nasal congestion. The pain of a cluster headaches is rooted in the **dilation** of blood vessels behind and around they eye which may be another autonomic response. Who knew that dilating blood vessels could be this painful but they are.

---

[8] https://www.ncbi.nlm.nih.gov/pmc/articles/PMC5909131/

Another very important component of cluster headaches is sudden release of histamine or serotonin in the body. Serotonin dilates blood vessels and there is some evidence that cluster headache sufferers have low serotonin.

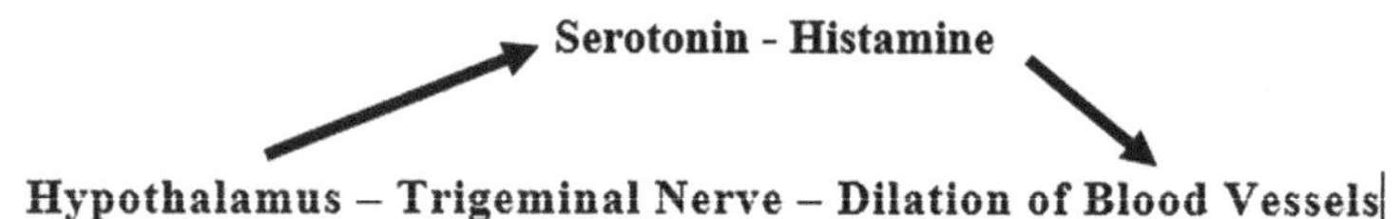

I am of the opinion that the serotonin / histamine component is a critical and often overlooked cause.

Serotonin is a chemical that carries messages between nerve cells in the brain and throughout your body. Serotonin plays a key role in such body functions as mood, sleep, digestion, nausea, wound healing, bone health, blood clotting and sexual desire.

Histamine is a compound which is released by cells in response to injury and in allergic and inflammatory reactions, causing contraction of smooth muscle and dilation of capillaries.

Is it Really Only A Headache?

Pain is the most curious phenomenon. To be human is to be acquainted with pain, be it emotional or physical. And only a fool would suggest that their pain is worse than another's, for pain is the most subjective of human feelings, and as they say, "we live in our heads".

Since that first cluster headache so many years ago I have often wondered how something this painful could not be doing some damage. As a young man I was sure that each attack was killing some brain cells. Pain is most often nature's way of telling us to get our hands off the hot stove for if we do not we will destroy tissue. Headaches can be caused by a tumor, a cerebral hemorrhage and a whole host of other serious maladies.

It turns out that cluster headaches are indeed essentially benign. They are not killing brain cells, there is no strong association with other diseases, and you have a very good chance of living a normal life span. One of the more controversial considerations regarding cluster headaches is co-morbidities. Cluster sufferers do indeed suffer from anxiety and depression at a disproportionate rate and this can lead to less than healthy lifestyle choices.[9]

Cluster headaches are bizarre and the fact that something this painful is indeed only a headache is equally and fittingly bizarre.

There is help and there is hope.

---

[9] Cluster Headache Tied to High Risk of Mental, Neurologic Disorders
Kelli Whitlock Burton
December 15, 2022 https://www.medscape.com/viewarticle/
985649?form=fpf#vp_2

References

Comizio, Christine. ***Ranking The Most Painful Medical Conditions***
April 13, 2023, at 4:38 p.m. **U.S. News and World Report**

Diana Yi-Ting Wei,[1,2] Jonathan Jia Yuan Ong,[1,3] and Peter James Goadsby[1,2] ***Cluster Headache: Epidemiology, Pathophysiology, Clinical Features, and*** Diagnosishttps://www.ncbi.nlm.nih.gov/pmc/articles/PMC5909131/

Headaches – cluster
https://www.mountsinai.org/health-library/report/headaches-cluster

Goadsby, Peter J., MD, PhD, Dsc, ***Treatment of Cluster Headache, American Headache Society,***
June 2018, https://americanheadachesociety.org/

Burton, Kelli Whitlock, ***Cluster Headache Tied to High Risk of Mental, Neurologic Disorders***
Kelli Whitlock Burton
December 15, 2022, https://www.medscape.com/viewarticle/985649?form=fpf#vp_2

Sharon A. Kandel; Pujyitha Mandiga.
Last update July 2023
National Institute of Health
National Library of Medicine
Cluster Headache
https://www.ncbi.nlm.nih.gov/books/NBK544241/

Resources

National Headache Foundation
https://headaches.org/

American Headache Society
https://americanheadachesociety.org/

Mayo Clinic
Cluster Headache
https://www.mayoclinic.org/diseases-conditions/
cluster-headache/diagnosis-treatment/drc-20352084

National Institute of Health
National Library of Medicine
Cluster Headache

https://www.ncbi.nlm.nih.gov/books/NBK544241/

Cleveland Clinic
Cluster Headaches
https://my.clevelandclinic.org/health/
diseases/5003-cluster-headaches

About the Author

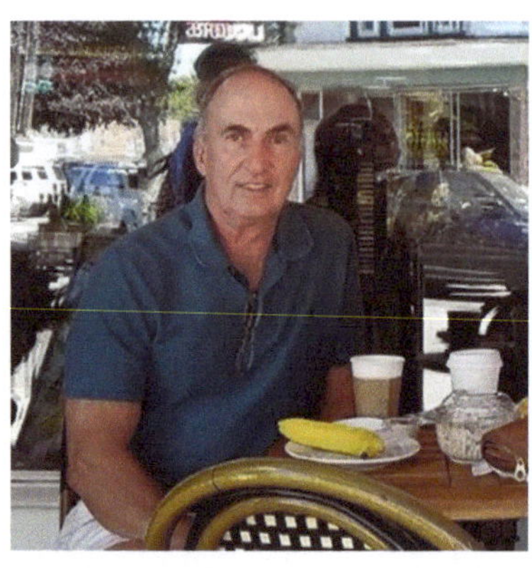

Jack Boyd is a happily retired and still working septua-genarian who is neither a medical Doctor nor a scientist. He is the retired Director of Quality Assurance for the Defense Contract Management Agency in Garden City NY who now works part time consulting and tutoring. He has an MBA from Dowling College and along with 2 years as a cadet at the U.S. Coast Guard Academy as an engineering major he holds a B.S. degree from St. Joseph's University in NY. His Graduate Record Exam qualified him for MENSA. He has 2 daughters and 2 grandchildren, and he divides his time between residences in Babylon Village and Southold on Long Island.

He likes to describe himself as a generalist who is capable of critical thinking. Most of his friends and associates would agree with this assessment.

He experienced his first cluster headache at the age of 21and after a lifetime of endurance, his reason for writing this handbook could be summarized as follows – **if not me, then who?**